Free Your **"SELF"** From Addiction!

By S. CASEY

Paperback ISBN: 979-8-9960711-0-4
eBook ISBN: 979-8-9960711-1-1

Table of Contents

Chapter 1

The start of this book is not going to be a lot about the history of addiction or the different types of addiction. If you're reading this book, you probably have a good idea about all of that. What you want to know is how to stop being an addict and get back to some form of control over your life. It doesn't matter if you spent the night in a dumpster, a vacant house, or woke up in a giant bed overlooking the ocean in Malibu—addiction happens to all types of people. Whether it be cocaine, pot, gambling, pornography, sex, heroin, fentanyl, or eating… addiction is addiction.

It doesn't matter if you're a new addict or you've been one for twenty years. If you have tried to quit a thousand times, have been through a dozen programs, and have not been able to stop permanently, you will have a way to get there by the end of this book—if you really want to and are open to looking at your addiction a different way. It won't require meetings, additional spending, or program sign-ups—just an open mind. It's very simple. If you can read, you're halfway there. I'll give you a hint: You are in a battle, and you may probably not even be aware of who you're fighting.

According to the National Aeronautics and Space Administration (NASA), they have a telescope that can see objects 13.5 billion light-years away (a beam of light traveling 5.88 trillion miles in one year) that is way, way out there! And so far, they have not found any sign of another Cleveland, Disneyland, or Starbucks. In all that vast emptiness, there is only this tiny planet called "Earth" with its 8.23 billion people spinning around this gigantic Sun every 365 days, and you're on it! Let that sink in for a bit.

Why are you here at this very moment in time, in this town or country, on this spinning planet? Why now? Why not during the American Revolution, or the Fall of the Roman Empire, or when Christopher Columbus first sailed to America? Why were you born into the family that you were in, or if you don't know your parents, why not? Why the school you attended or the job you may or may not have had? Why have all the life choices that you have made or the circumstances you have faced led you to this very moment in time? I bet that when you woke up this morning, you did not pay much attention to the fact that this might be the most important day of your life; that the choice you make after reading this book can and will determine your life's journey for all your years. Let's keep an open mind and move on.

Chapter 2

I want to tell you about a friend of mine, Michael, who is thirty-five and comes from a very wealthy family and wants for nothing. He is an only child who has always lived a privileged life and is accustomed to having things go his way. He is the CEO of a large international company and gets paid very, very well. When his parents passed away, from a horrendous automobile accident in Europe, he inherited a vast oceanfront estate in an exclusive summer beach town. Between Memorial Day and Labor Day, he would invite all his friends from the city for some very active weekend parties. These weekends became famous with lots of drugs, alcohol, and sex. People of all types would show up at these parties. In fact, so many people attended his parties; most of them he did not know, as they had come with guests. People would start showing up on Friday, and if everyone was gone by Monday morning, he didn't seem to mind. They slept wherever they could and brought their own alcohol and drugs. He provided the massive grounds, house, and music.

One Saturday in mid-June, he received a call from a friend asking if he could bring some people along.

And, of course, he said, "Yes, the more, the merrier." Two hours later, his friend arrived with three members of an outlaw motorcycle club, accompanied by their girlfriends. There was not much he could do as he had already invited them, and in a way, he thought it might even be cool to have members of a motorcycle gang at one of his famous summer parties. It would be the talk of the city.

The weekend was a great success, with the party lasting until Sunday afternoon, when most people started to leave. When Michael left for the city on Monday morning, the bikers were still at the pool house. That Wednesday, Michael received a call from the caretaker at the summer house, informing him that his motorcycle guests had not left and were still engaged in a lot of "partying." Michael told the caretaker he would come down the following day.

When Michael confronted the group, he explained that they would have to leave, but they were welcome to return the following weekend. They told Michael that they had no plans of leaving. Michael told them he would call the police, and they just laughed.

When the police arrived and heard Michael's account, they confronted the motorcycle group, who then produced a document resembling a contract. It stated that Michael had hired the group for the summer as an on-site security team and that they had a legally binding contract. After reviewing the agreement, the police informed Michael that it was a civil matter, and he would need to take it to court, as there was no further action they could take.

Michael was furious and could not believe what was happening. He wanted these people out of his pool house, and there was nothing he could do about it. He had lost all authority and control over his own property.

The motorcycle gang members did end up leaving the property when federal agents raided the estate on Labor Day weekend, arresting the "bikers" for drug dealing to the local beach community.

Michael's simple decision to allow something into his life ended with consequences that were never intended. The authority and control he thought he could exercise at will ended up being overridden by his original act of submission.

Let that sink in for a while.

Chapter 3

There always seems to be an opposite to something that shares the same sphere, not necessarily of equal measure. When a vacuum appears, the space will be filled by something —usually the opposite. Night…day, up…down, right…left, yin…yang, natural…spiritual, good…evil, God…Satan, etc., and so on. Some things can't be seen, but that doesn't mean they are not real. You can usually see their effects. The wind blows, the flag waves, and the ocean current sends the boat adrift. The electric current powers the light bulb. When there is balance, there is less chance of harm. Some, if not properly managed and balanced, can have devastating long-term consequences.

Let's look at the four pillars of power: Physical, Mental, Moral, and the highest and strongest, Spiritual. Physical, the least powerful, is based on the physical world protecting you or not, based on your "physical strength." This is the most primitive of the four. Next is Mental.

This is based on the information you have gained through life and the knowledge you have retained. Using your senses (sight, hearing, smell, taste, and touch) can trigger information that, with mental strength, can also protect you. The third pillar of strength is Moral, and it can also keep you protected in your daily life. And the last and most powerful is Spiritual. This is the one that 99 percent of humanity lacks and fails to utilize to its fullest potential for protection.

So, suppose you are an Olympic rower (Physical) who graduated from an Ivy League University (Mental) and comes from a well-respected, prominent family (Moral), but lacks a strong Spiritual connection. In that case, that vacuum will become a weakness and a lack of protection. And if you're not using all four pillars to their fullest potential, you allow a vacuum to be filled with something, because it always will.

You might think that you don't have a spiritual deficiency. You might be religious, or you might have regularly attended some form of church service, now or in the past. You might have even been baptized when you were three weeks old, but none of that matters…NOW. You have an addiction problem, and for some reason, none of that has protected you…WHY?

Appetite and authority are two words that say a lot about your current situation with addiction. Often, what starts for pleasure turns into pain. It's the very nature of addiction. One ends up needing more to get the previous pleasure that one got beforehand, taking one further into the addiction trap. One thinks they can easily stop but finds that their appetite becomes unsatisfied and uncontrollable. And the ability to stop, to say "no," becomes impossible to do. Why can't you say "no"? Is it because you are weak, you have this addiction gene in your DNA, you're a victim of society, or your spouse left you?

No, the real reason is, you did it yourself! Let me correct that, SELF did this to YOU. This thing called SELF has become the CEO of your life, and it is not your best friend. In fact, when it comes to YOU, your interests are not always SELF's interest. See, "self-interest" is not what you think it is. Neither is self-control, self-discovery, self-sufficiency, nor any of the other "selves" in the dictionary. It is strictly "SELF-FIRST"…YOU second. Let that sink in a bit.

What about the word "authority?" The dictionary defines it as the power to influence, control, or command. Do you really think you have much authority? People who are rich and famous think so, as do government officials. Police officers have authority, and judges do too. But how much authority do you really have? If you're an addict, you sure don't have authority or control over your own body. You might think you do, but how is that working for you? The truth is that addiction is a form of control—control that YOU have given away. But there are reinforcements to get it back, just waiting for your commands.

Imagine you were born in England in the 1400s during feudal times. There you were, living on a small farm that you did not own. The deal was that you could work your few acres, and whatever money you made, you gave half to the landowner. You were a free person, not under the landowner's authority. If something were to happen to you on the way to the marketplace, if you were robbed or beaten, you would be on your own. The landowner was not responsible for providing any form of safety, support, or protection. The robbers and thieves along the road would recognize you as a peon, an easy target.

But suppose you were under a different landowner, one who owned many acres and employed many farmers to work on his land. He also had a group of knights who protected his castle and all the people on his land. Then, when you took your goods to market to sell, the robbers would know you were under the authority of the landowner with the knights and would grant you safe passage.

The same person, but one with protection. Where are your knights?

Chapter 4

Let's get to the heart of the matter…SELF. You're really made up of four components: SELF, your SPIRIT, your SOUL, and YOU. At a certain point in the future, all four are going to leave the vessel they are currently contained in—your body.

You are going to stop breathing, your heart will arrest, and you will cease to exist in this form. You might be very aware of one of these, but perhaps not so much of the other three. Maybe you have religious beliefs, or you have some awareness of "something else" — a "higher power" — in your life; but if you're like most people, you've given 99.9 percent of your attention to one of these, and very little to the other three. You are very aware of its power: As you ask, "Why couldn't I control my SELF? I'm going to do it by my SELF." Here's a question: If mankind has evolved, why does SELF put YOU in situations that are harmful to YOU? By now, SELF should be protecting the other three: your SPIRIT, your

SOUL, and YOU, but it doesn't. It has its own agenda, it has its own self-interest, and it may or may not always have your best interest.

Like my friend with the summer house, SELF likes to have a good time—sometimes. And SELF will do things without asking YOUR permission. You might ask, aren't SELF and YOU both the same? They're not!

YOU, as owner of "Your Castle," have, over time, given all authority and power to SELF and have let your SPIRIT, your SOUL, and YOU take a backseat to the decisions and direction of your life's journey. In fact, you might not even be aware of the other three at all. When it comes to making a life decision, your SELF is so strong, it will always get its way. In fact, if YOU get a "sense" that your decision might be wrong, your SELF will play the self-confident and self-assured card to stay in control. SELF does not want any self-governance of "itself"! That would be self-defeating.

You may be saying, I know about SELF, but not so much about my SPIRIT and my SOUL. And that's where SELF wants to leave it. See,

SELF is sitting on the throne in "Your Castle" and is running things like it has all the authority, leaving your SPIRIT with no say at all, as YOU stand by and let this happen. You might "feel" like something is going on. Still, you blame all your bad decisions on your inability to make good decisions for whatever reason: you're weak or have a bad marriage, heredity, and so on, never knowing that SELF is the real cause.

Let's go back to why you're here: …What is the primary purpose of this thing we call life? As I said at the beginning of this book, freeing you from addiction is really the easiest part; how we get there is going to require YOU (not SELF) to have an open mind and for some to answer a few difficult questions.

The first question to answer is: Do you believe in some form of a "higher power?"

You don't have to be religious; you need some curiosity about spirituality. Maybe you don't spend much time thinking about why you're on this planet, or what happens after "you pass on." You may even be an atheist—but, by the time you get through with this book, you will have a very clear knowledge of why you're here. It will be up to YOU to acknowledge and accept it or not—because YOU have "self-will."

Chapter 5

Let's go back to the summer house and my friend. He allowed some members of a motor-cycle gang onto his property, but they refused to leave. That's what SELF did to YOU!

In the Spirit World, the one you can't see, but is all around us—when you took that first snort of cocaine at the company sales convention, YOU thought it would only be a one-time thing. In fact, SELF convinced YOU that it would be a one-time thing. The difference between never trying something and trying it 100 times is that one time. YOU, without knowing it, permitted an outside source to enter "Your Castle," and in that process, gave up all authority to tell it to leave.

In the Bible, spirits are mentioned hundreds of times. There are good spirits and evil spirits, such as the "Spirit of Addiction" and the "Spirit of Bondage." Once you let your SELF make that decision to snort the cocaine, your actions and verbal commands permit those spirits to enter

"Your Castle." Just like the motorcycle gang members, those spirits won't leave.

Now you know who you're fighting against; the question is, why? To get the answer, we must first look to the Bible and the "Garden of Eden." I hear you saying, "What does that have to do with my addiction?" but it all starts with that apple tree. From the beginning, mankind was meant to have a personal relationship with its "Creator." In fact, Adam and God would often walk in the Garden and talk. Then Satan tricked Eve into eating the apple, which God had commanded them not to do. Whether it was an apple, a pear, or a banana, it was a symbol of disobedience to God's command, and the start of all the world's problems. After Adam ate the apple, they hid from God in the garden. One day, God called for Adam, and Adam, hiding in the bushes, replied that he was naked. God asked, "Who told you that you are naked?" This was the start of man's "self-consciousness." Humanity could never have the "living personal relationship" with God, as had been planned initially, and it's where your very problem with SELF began. It's part of your nature, and you're born with it: ask any mother as she watches her three-month-old baby tossing toys out of the crib.

And SELF only gets stronger every day—if YOU let it!

Chapter 6

So, let's go back to the question: Why are you here? Why are your circumstances the way they are? Do you really think you are entirely in control of your life? The people you meet, the place you are in, are all based on what you did? Or is there something else going on that you can't see, and don't even know exists?

At the beginning of the Bible are two statements that are very important to understand your addiction. The first: "God created man in His image." God is the Creator. You were born to "create." To build, design, and make—be it music, buildings, pies, or whatever, but to create what God has put as talents in your body for His Kingdom, not yours. But SELF doesn't see it that way. SELF wants what it wants. It has its own "self-interest," not God's or yours.

The second important statement that God said in creating the world was, "Let there be light." God spoke those words, and the critical part of creating is being verbal. God did not think, "Let there be light." He spoke it. Words that come out of your mouth let the Universe put those actions into place, and what you say has consequences. It gives the Universe authority to create what you have commanded.

If your SELF says, "Let's get high," and YOU don't think that's a good idea, but SELF convinces YOU that it's just this one time, and your mouth opens and says, "Yeah, I'll take a snort." YOU have just given the go-ahead for Satan to send the "Spirit of Addiction," and the "Spirit of Bondage" to take up permanent residence in "Your Castle." Understand this: Satan cannot put you under his control unless YOU permit him. And addiction is a form of control. You might not know you're doing that, but that's what you've done. Like my friend's summer house and the motorcycle gang members, you now have some permanent unwanted "guests" in "Your Castle."

Because you are not aware of your new "friends," you're also not aware of how to get rid of them. SELF is of no use as it has no power or authority to remove them. You might ask: "Why is this going on?" The answer is much more complicated than the destruction of your life. Since the fall in the "Garden," Satan has been lying to mankind, and he will lie to YOU…through SELF (self-deception) to keep you from claiming what is rightfully yours, your inheritance and a personal relationship with GOD, here on Earth, before you go to Heaven.

Chapter 7

My friend, Bill, had an uncle, with whom he was not very close, who lived in Texas. After retiring from thirty years of replacing roofs on the East Coast, Bill decided to get a small travel trailer and take a cross-country vacation. He had worked hard all his life and had never taken any time off; he couldn't afford to. Upon arriving in Texas, he visited the company his uncle owned. He discovered that his uncle had passed away five years earlier, leaving him the company, which was now valued at over ten million dollars. He questioned why no one had contacted him. They replied that the "will" prevented it, as his uncle only wanted to give Bill the company if he showed up.

That's kind of where you're at now. You have an inheritance, power, and authority worth more than money, but you're not even aware of it, nor how to claim it. And to make matters even worse, Satan will do everything he can to be sure you never do. In fact, Satan will ruin your life so severely that SELF will convince YOU that there is no chance of hope—but that too is a lie.

You're probably aware of solids, liquids, and gases. You can see two of them, but the third — gases — are sometimes impossible to see. You can't see the wind, but you can see the effects of the wind— "trees and grass blowing in the wind." The "Spirit World" is like that. You can't see the "Spirit of Addiction" or the "Spirit of Bondage," but you can see the damage it causes and the control it has on people. And like the Bible mentions hundreds of times, spirits and demons are real.

So, the question is, now that you know who you're fighting against, what can you do about it? Well, we need to go back to the Garden of Eden. Since then, mankind has tried through prayer, works, and sacrifices to regain what it has lost—a personal relationship with God—but has consistently failed to do so. Finally, God has provided a way. All a person needs to do is accept the gift of acknowledgment. It requires something so simple, yet difficult. It requires YOU to remove SELF from the throne of "Your Castle" and replace it with its rightful owner.

Doesn't matter if you're Jewish, Buddhist, Muslim, or any other religion; it's the same GOD, and He has made it known that He wants to have a personal relationship with YOU, and the only way to do that is to make JESUS your LORD and SAVIOR.

Once those words come out of your mouth, you kick SELF off the throne of "Your Castle" and put GOD in His rightful place.

You become "BORN AGAIN." You get a "NEW HEART." You are now a "NEW CREATURE" different than before, distinct from the rest, with the power and authority of a PRIEST and a KING, to be used to bring glory to HIS KINGDOM. And, as you are now a "CHILD OF GOD," you now have the power to claim your inheritance. In God's EYES, you are a "NEW PERSON," and because you are, HE can now start to have that personal relationship with you and put the HOLY SPIRIT into your life to guide you on your life's journey NOW—BEFORE you go to Heaven.

You now have someone who has the authority to kick out the "Spirit of Addiction" and the

"Spirit of Bondage" who have been living in "Your Castle," sitting on your couch, watching TV, drinking beer, and eating chips just waiting for the opportunity to fuel your addiction.

Chapter 8

Remember the Four Pillars of Power: Physical, Mental, Moral, and Spiritual? Now, here is the problem you face. You live in a physical world, dealing with a physical problem, but the solution for your addiction is on the spiritual side of your life. Recognize this and you're halfway there. The world will allow you to talk about a god anytime. They will even acknowledge there might be a god, but Satan will do everything he can to stop you from ever mentioning the name Jesus or for you to accept Him as your Lord and Savior. He will trick you into "12-step programs" that are supposed to cure your addictions and that even acknowledge a "higher power." The problem with those programs is that they have no authority to remove the "Spirit of Addiction" and the "Spirit of Bondage" from "Your Castle." In fact, every time you start one of their meetings, they remind you of what you still are: "Hi, my name is Jim, I'm a cocaine addict." "Hi Jim!"

When you accept Jesus, you are "BORN AGAIN," you are a "NEW CREATURE," your past is forgotten in God's eyes, your slate is wiped clean, and you are given a new start. Not on anything you have done, like giving money to a church, or by saying prayers five times a day, or even trying to be a good person, but only by opening your mouth and accepting JESUS as your Lord and Savior. When that happens, God moves into "Your Castle" and will immediately start to sweep out those spirits "FOREVER," and Satan will do everything he can to make sure that doesn't happen.

As I stated at the beginning of this book, this was not really about addiction; it's about bondage and control. And it's not a "religious" book, it is a "spiritual" book. It doesn't matter if you're Jewish, Muslim, Christian, Hindu, or Buddhist; when you accept Jesus into your life, you now have a real living "GOD" inside of you, ready to guide your life to happiness, joy, and peace. He will not let you continue to be under the bondage of spirits that will harm you. As Jesus said,

"I have come to set you free. I come so you can have life more abundantly."

Look at it this way, once a wealthy man offered a younger man this opportunity: "I cannot travel, so I would like to see the world through your eyes. Come to the train station tomorrow at 10:00 a.m. and do not bring anything. In fact, leave everything you own behind; do not even bring a change of clothes or any money. When you arrive at the station, please mention my name at the office, and they will provide you with a ticket. Once you board the train, you will be on the best journey of your life, meant for you to take. Everything will be provided for you if you follow the instructions that I will provide along the way. Your best interest will always be mine to give you." That is what God wants you to do: Make Jesus your Lord and Savior.

That's where you're at now. If you woke up this morning in a dumpster, a cheap motel room, or spent the night under a bridge, if you've ruined your life, destroyed your family, or lost your job, it's not too late. It can all turn around.

Addiction is a "spiritual attack of bondage and control" against the very existence of your life NOW, and when you pass. It doesn't have to be that way. God wants to have that "personal relationship" you were meant to have, and Jesus is God's redemption plan to do it. But you have "Self-will," and God will not force YOU.

God is a Spirit, and you need to let YOUR SPIRIT have that relationship with Him. It's now up to YOU to remove SELF from continuing to control your life…—it's that simple. In fact, the most essential words in the Bible that Jesus spoke were "Deny Self and Follow Me."

Chapter 9

I have a friend who recently invited me over to his house for a cookout. As we were sitting outside, his dog came out of the house and started to chase his tail—around and around and around he went, never catching it. I told my friend that this type of behavior would probably stop as the dog gets older and his tail grows out. He just laughed and said he had been cutting the dog's tail for some time and that it was fun to watch.

Is that what is happening to you? Satan will do everything he can to keep you from claiming what is rightfully yours: an inheritance and a personal relationship with God. Satan will use whatever he has to keep you under his control, and addiction is one way to do it. If you do not learn about the battle you're in and why, you will always be chasing your tail in a never-ending quest to get freed from addiction. You are now at that crossroad.

So, let's summarize your problem. You're in a game with two players, and you are the prize.

This is a "spiritual battle" that has ramifications that will last for eternity. One player wants to ruin your life, and addiction is part of that. The other player wants to set you free and have a loving relationship with you now and forever. One will win and one will lose, and you have up until your last breath when the "game" is over.

Satan is a liar and will use your emotions to trick you. He will use SELF and "addiction" to control you so that the words, "I make Jesus my Lord and Savior," never come out of your mouth. When that happens, it's over for him. Remember, Satan has no control, power, or authority over you unless YOU give it to him, whether you know it or not. He also knows that SELF does not always have your best interests and can be easily tricked. YOU are the one who decides the "winner" of this game, your destiny, and if you want to be FREED FROM ADDICTION.

You are now at your "GARDEN OF EDEN MOMENT." Instead of Adam, it's YOU. Instead of the apple, it's SELF. Instead of taking, it's giving. Instead of selfishness, it's selfless. Instead of Satan telling you "Yes," he's now telling you

"No." And instead of YOU pushing God away, you're pulling Him toward YOU. Instead of then, it's NOW!

This is the time to take SELF off the throne of "Your Castle" and put the One who has absolute authority, that even Satan, with his "Spirit of Addiction" and "Spirit of Bondage" must obey—and that is JESUS!

WARNING: SELF will now start to work on YOU to try to convince YOU that this is too far-fetched, and this is not the time for you to get "religious." That, before you got your addiction problem, you might have attended some "religious service"—you might even belong to a church now—and you might even have been baptized when you were three months old. None of that matters now, or even what religion you are, if you've never said the words, "I make Jesus my Lord and Savior." It must verbally come out of your mouth to set the Universe in motion.

And if SELF is still telling YOU this is too hard to believe, remember this: That you are one of 8.23 billion "human beings" on this planet, spinning around a giant fireball called the Sun, in a vast emptiness of space, at this very moment in time.

If you're now ready to take back control of your life, your rightful inheritance, power, and authority, and experience the life you were meant to have, please accept His offer. The following few pages will guide you on how to go about that—it's that simple!

Also, if you're reading this book because you have a loved one who has an addiction problem and you want to help, please read Addendum 3 now.

Chapter 10

No matter where you are right now—outside, in a closet, or in a dumpster—look up to Heaven and with palms pointing upward, say: "Heavenly Father, forgive me of my sins. Please change my life. I make Jesus my Lord and Savior. Fill me with the Holy Spirit and remove the "Spirit of Addiction" and the "Spirit of Bondage" from my life forever. I ask this in Jesus' name, Amen."

It's that simple! Continue living the life you have right now and LET GOD DO HIS THING! SELF will want to "do something" to try and "Help Him." Don't do that. It's not your strength that will "set you free from addiction," but Jesus'. You don't need to do anything more; you did what was necessary when you made Jesus your Lord.

When you did that, you kicked SELF off the throne of "Your Castle," and you made Satan the "big loser." In God's eyes, you became "Born Again," and you set the Universe into action, and "tens of thousands of Angels" blew their trumpets in celebration! The Holy Spirit moved into "Your Castle," and now you have the Holy Spirit inside of you. "Your Castle" is now a "Temple" with Jesus on the throne. The spirits that have held you in bondage will be gone, and your appetite for your addiction will begin to disappear over time. You will still be tempted, and you WILL have setbacks—when you do, acknowledge that in prayer, and ask for forgiveness. God will forgive you and continue to guide you into new situations and opportunities that will change your life. Understand that God does not need your help; He needs your belief and trust! "Stand still and wait upon the Lord." It means just that.

What you can do is start each day by giving thanks. "Heavenly Father, thank you for this day, thank you for the blessings I have and the ones that are on their way. Thank you for being my God, for giving me a new heart, and freeing me of the 'Spirit of Addiction' and the 'Spirit of Bondage' from my life forever. I ask this in Jesus' name, Amen."

You are now beginning a personal living relationship with the Creator of the Universe that is now in "Your Temple." Throughout the day, try to become "aware" of that, and give thanks to Jesus on any "little" blessing that will start to come your way. Whether it's finding a penny on the sidewalk, a parking spot up front, or avoiding a pothole—thank Him. As you become more attuned to your "spiritual side," you will start to get a "feeling" about people, places, and things that might not be good for you. This is the Holy Spirit trying to "guide" you to protection. You will then "naturally" start to avoid those situations that could tempt you, and the Holy Spirit will give you the strength to do that.

Some last thoughts—on your FREEDOM. As they say, "Freedom is not Free," but the price to get you out of bondage has been paid by someone else, and that someone is Jesus.

Give thanks for that every day.

The shackles have been removed. You are a "New Person" with a "New Heart," and a living God inside of you—with the power, authority, and inheritance that comes with that. Your job is to "Believe and Trust." Jesus will do the rest—guaranteed!

Addendum 1

Everyday Tips: If you really want to improve your "Physical" pillar of power, you might decide to get healthy and strong. You might spend more time in the gym and pay closer attention to what you eat. Your results would depend on your "personal daily commitment."

You would have to do the same if you wanted to improve your "Spiritual" pillar of power. Here are a few tips you can use throughout the day to accomplish that.

Start each day with prayer: "Heavenly Father, thank you for this day, thank you for the blessings I have and the ones that are on the way. Free me from all addictions and change my life. I ask this in Jesus' name, Amen."

End each day with a prayer: "Heavenly Father, forgive me for any sins that I have committed this day, in thought or in action, wipe my slate clean and let me start again. Please free me from all addictions and change my life. I ask this in Jesus' name, Amen."

Start reading the Bible: You will now be able to understand it in ways that were previously impossible to you. God is a Spirit and is now able to communicate with your Spirit. You will now be able to understand and, in a way, "hear" what He has to say. You will also be able to claim the hundreds of promises that God has provided for you. Promises like prosperity, good health, joy, peace, protection, and more.

If one is in a relationship, one usually "talks things over" with each other before taking action. A husband would never bring home a $100,000 motor home without "talking it over" with his wife first. You are now in a "Personal Relationship" with God. If you need to make a decision, "no matter how small," run it by Him first—remember, He is your Lord. Here's the good part: you can't go wrong when you do this. He wants to be a part of your life, and He will always make sure things "turn out OK" when you involve Him from the beginning.

Also, understand this: God is no longer outside of you but is now inside of you. You no longer need to go to buildings with "stained glass" windows, "marble floors," or "statues of saints" to visit and speak with God. He's right inside of you every moment of the day. So, try to live with this in mind.

Addendum 2

<u>Some Biblical promises for you to claim:</u>

Jesus said, "<u>I am the way</u>, and the truth, and the life. No one comes to the Father except through Me."

Whoever is <u>a believer</u> in Christ is a <u>new creation</u>.

I will give you a <u>new heart</u> and put a <u>new spirit </u>within you. You are <u>God's temple,</u> and God's Spirit <u>dwells in you</u>.

But the <u>Lord is faithful</u>, and He will <u>strength-en you</u> and <u>protect you</u> from the evil one.

Be on your guard and stay awake. Your enemy, the devil, is like a roaring lion, sneaking around to find someone to attack.

For He will order His angels to <u>protect you</u> in all you do.

Because <u>the One who is in you is greater</u> than the one who is in the world.

And Jesus said, "<u>All authority</u> in heaven and on earth has been given to Me."

Commit everything you do to the LORD. <u>Trust Him</u>, and He will help you.

I can do all things <u>through Christ,</u> which strengthen me.

Addendum 3

If you bought this book because you have a loved one or friend who has an addiction problem, there are two ways you can help them. One is to give them this book. If you don't know where they are, then that won't work. The second way will require more "conviction to help" than you may or may not have. You will have to kick "Self" off the throne in "Your Castle" and put Jesus on it.

In doing this, you will get back the authority, power, and inheritance that you can use to act as an INTERCESSOR for your loved one. Being BORN AGAIN, you now have access to the Creator of the World that only a "Child of God" has. And through prayer each day, you can MEDIATE and PETITION on behalf of your loved one in Jesus' name and KNOW that He will do what He has promised.

"Heavenly Father, I ask for forgiveness of my sins. I make Jesus my Lord and Savior. Please remove the "Spirit of Addiction" and the "Spirit of Bondage" from (add name) and change his/her life forever. I ask this in Jesus' name, Amen."

As mentioned before, SELF is very selfish and does not want to give up its authority. Are YOU willing to take SELF off the throne to get Freedom from Bondage and Addiction for a loved one? This is really your "Garden of Eden" moment. It's that simple!

Addendum 4

YOU (1) versus SELF (198)

YOU
SELF
Self-abandonment, Self-abasement, Self-abnegation, Self-absorption, Self-abuse, Self-accusation, Self-acting, Self-actualization, Self-addressed, Self-adhesive, Self-adjusting, Self-admiration, Self-advancement, Self-advertisement, Self-advocacy, Self-affirmation, Self-aggrandizement, Self-alienation, Self-aligning, Self-analysis, Self-annihilation, Self-appointed, Self-approbation, Self-approval, Self-assembly, Self-assertion, Self-assessment, Self-assurance, Self-awareness, Self-betrayal, Self-canceling, Self-censorship, Self-centered, Self-cleaning, Self-closing, Self-colored, Self-compatible, Self-conceit, Self-concept, Self-condemnation, Self-confessed, Self-confidence, Self-congratulation, Self-conscious, Self-consistent, Self-contained,

Self-contempt, Self-control, Self-correcting, Self-created, Self-critical, Self-deception, Self-defeating, Self-defense, Self-definition, Self-delight, Self-delusion, Self-denial, Self-dependence, Self-deprecating, Self-despair, Self-destroying, Self-destruct, Self-determination, Self-development, Self-devotion, Self-directed, Self-discipline, Self-discovery, Self-disgust, Self-doubt, Self-dramatization, Self-educated, Self-effacing, Self-employed, Self-enclosed, Self-esteem, Self-evaluation, Self-evident, Self-examination, Self-excited, Self-existent, Self-explanatory, Self-expression, Self-faced, Self-feeder, Self-fertile, Self-financing, Self-flagellation, Self-flattery, Self-forgetful, Self-fulfilling, Self-generating, Self-glorification, Self-government, Self-gravitation, Self-hatred, Self-heal, Self-help, Selfhood, Self-identification, Self-identity, Selfie, Self-image, Self-immolation, Self-importance, Self-imposed, Self-improvement, Self-incompatible, Self-induced, Self-indulgence, Self-inflicted, Self-insurance, Self-interest, Self-involved,

Selfish, Self-justification, Self-knowledge, Selfless, Self-limiting, Self-liquidating, Self-loading, Self-locking, Self-love, Self-made, Self-management, Self-mastery, Self-mate, Self-mocking, Self-mortification, Self-motion, Self-motivated, Self-murder, Self-mutilation, Self-neglect, Selfless, Self-opinionated, Self-parody, Self-perpetuating, Self-pity, Self-policing, Self-pollination, Self-portrait, Self-possessed, Self-praise, Self-preservation, Self-proclaimed, Self-propelled, Self-propagating, Self-protection, Self-realization, Self-referential, Self-reflection, Self-regard, Self-regulating, Self-reliance, Self-renewal, Self-renunciation, Self-reproach, Self-respecting, Self-restraint, Self-revealing, Self-righteous, Self-righting, Self-rising, Self-rule, Self-sacrifice, Self-same, Self-satisfied, Self-sealing, Self-seed, Self-seeking, Self-selection, Self-serving, Self-similar, Self-slaughter, Self-sow, Self-starter, Self-sterile, Self-stick, Self-stimulation, Self-styled, Self-subsistence, Self-sufficient, Self-suggestion, Self-supporting, Self-surrender, Self-sustaining,

Self-system, Self-tapping, Self-taught, Self-timer, Self-torture, Self-transcendence, Self-understanding, Self-willed, Self-winding, Self-worth.

Jesus said, "Deny Self and Follow Me."